# June 2018

# HOPE

After Brain Injury

**HOPE**
MAGAZINE

*"Supporting the
Brain Injury Community"*

# Welcome



## HOPE MAGAZINE

*Serving the Brain Injury Community*

### June 2018

**Publisher**
David A. Grant

**Editor**
Sarah Grant

### Contributing Writers
Tobie-Lynn Andrade
David A. Grant
Ric Johnson
Christine Lawrence
Norma Myers
Rosemary Rawlins
Ted Stachulski
Donavan Vliet

*FREE subscriptions at
www.HopeAfterBrainInjury.com*



Welcome to the June 2018 issue of HOPE Magazine!

This month's issue of HOPE Magazine features stories that have a common theme. You will read about survivors, and those who love them, who have learned to adapt and change after brain injury.

Those who face brain injury firsthand can speak to the major life changes that come with such a life-altering event. Personalities often change, family dynamics change, relationships change, employment status changes (or disappears). The list goes on.

Somehow, against seemingly insurmountable odds, we find our way by learning to embrace the changes and begin our lives anew. The journey is not an easy one, but it is possible. A meaningful life after brain injury is a reality for so many within our community.

A few butterflies grace the pages of our June issue, a living example of change. They are a perfect symbol of new life as they learn to soar as the new creatures they have become.

And so it is my wish for you today – that you are able to walk through the darkness, and emerge with wings to fly.

Peace,

David A. Grant
*Publisher*

# Contents




2   Publishers Introduction

4   Moving with a Brain Injury

9   One More Day

12  Moving Forward

15  Changing Roles

18  The Many Faces of Brain Injury and Grief

23  The Only Normal I Know

28  Grasp the Life Ring

29  Overlooked Vision Problems

37  News & Views


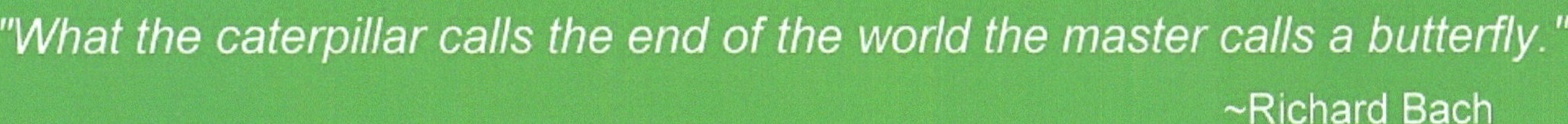

*"What the caterpillar calls the end of the world the master calls a butterfly."*

~Richard Bach

# Moving with a Brain Injury

## By Tobie-Lynn Andrade

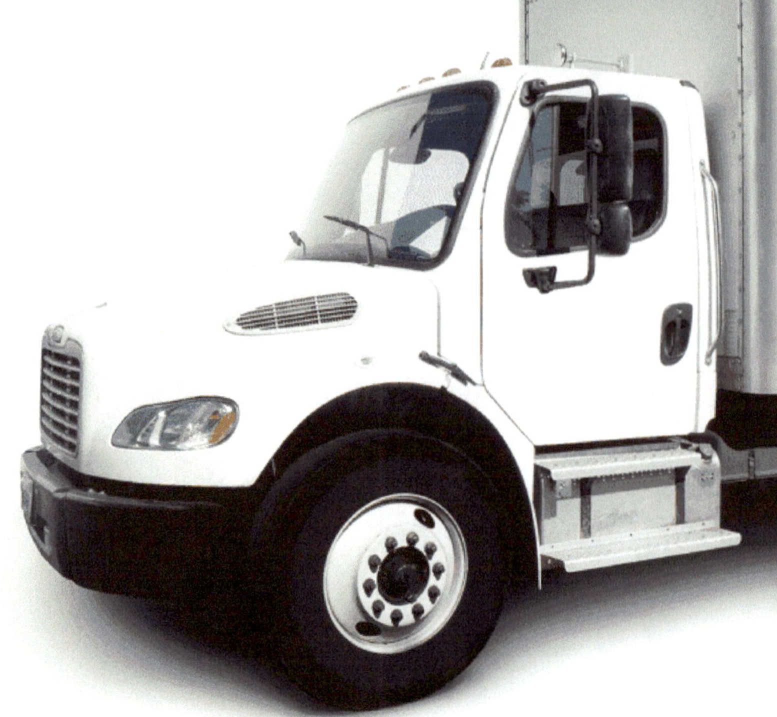

Moving is one of the most stressful life tasks we do. Even prior to my brain injury, it was not a task that I enjoyed, and I know we stayed in some rentals longer than we should have. This was simply because I did not want to move. It is not that the result is not usually a good one. Most people choose to move to a larger or smaller home for life reasons, perhaps a change of city due to employment opportunities or just because you have found your dream home.

I am fortunate to have moved a lot. In the last seventeen years we have moved our home address thirteen times and my husband's business four times. I do not really enjoy the process though I am now very efficient at moving from all the practice I have had.

> "In less than four weeks, we went from finding out we were moving to finding a new home and actually moving."

I am currently in the middle of a move not by choice. In less than four weeks, we went from finding out we were moving to finding a new home and actually moving. I have relied on my past moving experiences. The organizational tips I am sharing have helped our moves go smoothly since my brain injury five years ago. These are the things I find most useful when we move.

**Know your new place.** Take photos and measurements so you have an idea of what furniture and fixings you want to put in the new rooms. Remember to check the window sizes in case you need coverings. Having sizes on hand before you move makes it easier. I take pictures of the rooms and have a pad and paper with me when we look at the new place, so I can draw a quick diagram of the rooms showing where windows are as well as closets/electrical outlets and a note if there is ceiling light or not.

**Purge as you pack.** If there are things that you are not using, this is a great time to get rid of them. I usually have a few piles or boxes for purging. Some to donate to local charities and some go to family.

**Take photos.** Make sure you take photos of your new home while it is still empty - especially if you are a renter you know what condition the home was in when you got it. If buying and upgrading you can see what the home looked like before you enhanced it. Also take photos of things like the back of your TV or stereo unit so you know where the plugs go for setting it up again after you move. Take photos of your curio or china cabinets to recall how you had your items displayed, it takes the guesswork out of putting them back together once you move and lessens the number of decisions you have to make.

**Be organized when packing.** I use a lot of Rubbermaid bins. We learned the hard way that not all garages or basements are dry. Also, if you have items that you are storing and not using right away, plastic totes are good for stacking and storing items, like Christmas decorations, long term without damaging them. Label what will go into storage, and where it is to be stored clearly. This is so your Christmas globes end up under the basement stairs where you want them and not in the linen closet.

**Label everything.** I channel my inner Sheldon from the Big Bang Theory. I have a label maker and use it a lot when we move. I have the TV unit set up with all the cords labelled so I know where the cords go once

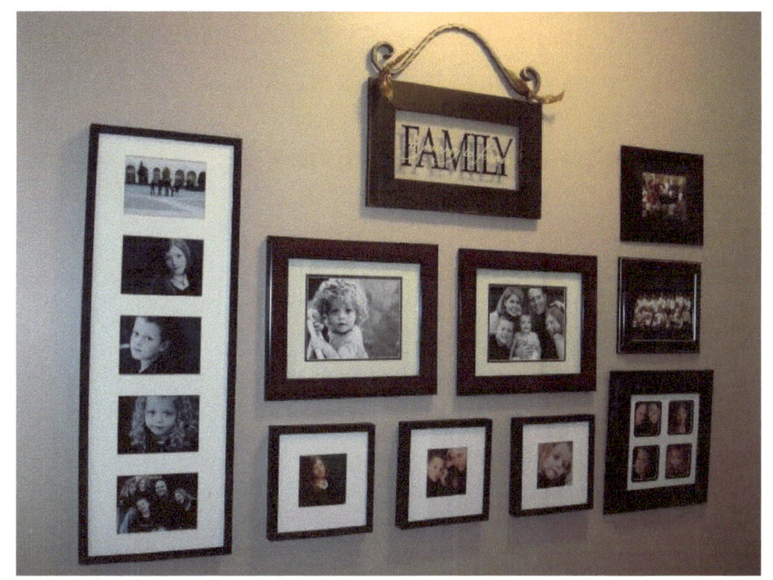

we set it up again. I not only put them on the back of the TV itself, but I have the plugs labelled where they go into the power bar. While I am packing boxes, I also label them. I use recipe or Index cards to write down what I am putting into the box. I then leave that card on the inside of the box so when I open it I know exactly what is in there. On the outside of the box, I put a less detailed label showing where I want it to go. "KITCHEN," and a basic description of what is inside it, "EVERYDAY DISHES" for example.

**Pack similar items together when possible.** This seems obvious, but once you have six rooms started and fourteen half-packed boxes, it is easy to start throwing things in wherever they fit. Try to keep rooms together where possible, or if you have collectibles around your home that fit together, pack them together. It's much easier to decide where to place that box in your new home if it's not mixed between several rooms or collections.

**Stack packed boxes according to which rooms they will go into whenever possible.** This makes it easier on everyone if this can happen. Personally, I try to pack boxes and put them into closets during the moving process. Off-season clothes and such are usually in the bedroom anyway, but keeping all the master bedroom items in your room makes it simple.

**Wrap and label your furniture.** We found that plastic wrap can be our friend, but not my husband's friend - he gets dizzy wrapping furniture. It has saved on the amount of scratches and dings our furniture gets. If you have particularly fragile or antique pieces, using pool noodles on the corners or edges helps as well. We have lots of old towels and blankets to cover furniture with and then we wrap the plastic wrap around it.

**Label the rooms on move day.** Some rooms seem obvious, but I have put signs on doors to indicate "kid's bathroom" or "master bedroom" when questions occur. I also put post-it notes on cupboard doors to show where I want my everyday dishes and cutlery, and which closet will be designated linens.  If I have a designated spot for a cabinet or piece of furniture I also put a sign or note on the wall where I want it placed. The less rearranging you can do after the initial move, the better.

**Make lists**. Keep your lists in obvious sight so that you and others know what needs doing.

When my parents come to help pack, my mom breezes through the kitchen and dining rooms, carefully wrapping the glassware while dad does the high shelves and taking down wall hangings. Know what your strengths are, as well as those of your packing team. I would not let my husband pack the fragile boxes. I don't try to pack or move his heavy research books.

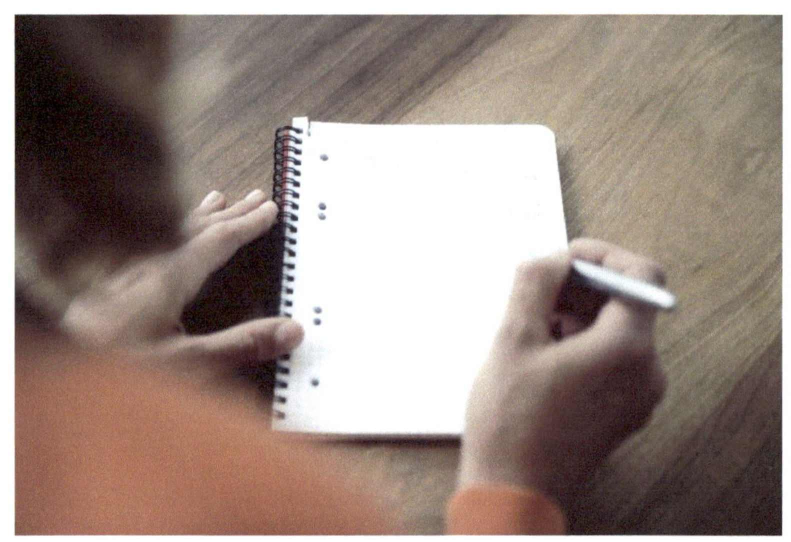

**Clean as you go.** I like to leave my home as clean as possible, but there is so much to do on the actual move day that I do not want to waste my time washing cupboards or windows. I slowly move through cupboards purging, packing and cleaning. Our current home has a huge bathroom vanity with lots of drawers. I empty one drawer at a time, clean it and reorganize it with what needs to be left out until the move. Come moving day, once I empty the drawer, it has already been cleaned and I just need to pick out the stray hairpins, but all the major cleaning is done.

**Go in stages**. Figure out what you need right up until you move. Your daily hygiene products, for example, will likely stay in the shower until the day you move. I pack my collectibles near the start of the move as they aren't essential to everyday life. You can do each room in stages as well. I pack my large holiday dishes early on. Anyone who knows me knows there is little chance of home cooked meals during a move, let alone large turkey dinners.

**Get Help**. Moving is not a foolproof process. Consider all the companies who thrive during this chaos by offering moving, packing, organizing services. If it is within your budget and out of your means to pack or organize, get help from the professionals. Not everyone moves with a U-Haul and family help. That said, use whatever help is available to you, and ask for more when needed. You would be surprised how simple it can go with some extra hands. Make sure that the people helping you know your process for packing, labelling, organizing and storing items before and during the move.

**On the big day, have a director or two.** It does not have to be you, but make sure someone is in charge of things at the old house as well as the new house. Our move is a local one, so our crew of family will be bouncing back and forth between both houses. It is a good idea to have a plan in place for physically moving. I like to get one room clear at a time. This way, while the sons and husband are moving the furniture, mom and I can make sure closets and drawers and cupboards are empty and clean.

> "At the new house, we have someone double-checking items and where they go, so that things end up in the right rooms."

We also sweep or vacuum that room and then shut the door until the final walk through so we know it is done. At the new house, we have someone double-checking items and where they go, so that things end up in the right rooms. Having the labels on the boxes and doors and walls helps in case you have a large group or complex move to make sure that everyone can see where things go.

**Do a final walk through of the old house**. As renters, we always do this. We also take photos in case there are any questions of damage or how the unit was left. We have the photos to compare from when we moved in to when we moved out.

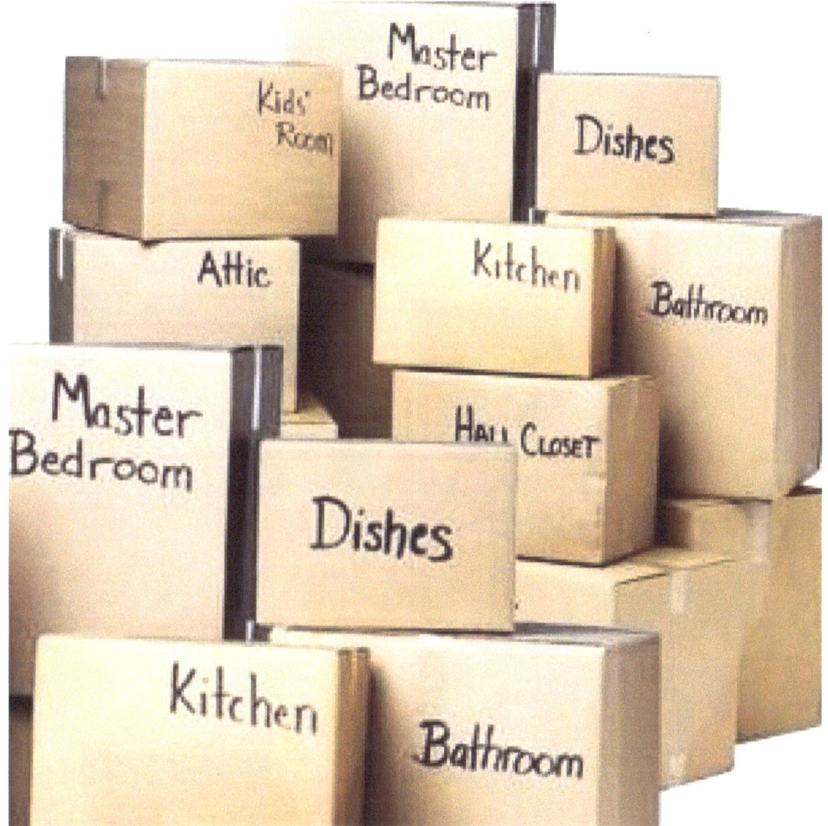


I usually email myself the pictures when we move in so that when we move out, I can refer to them. I also keep all the lease and payment information in same email file. It also makes it simple to check and be sure you haven't left anything behind and to make sure all is clean when you hand over the keys.

Keep calm and pace yourself. Use every tool in your box to keep calm, organized, and healthy. You know yourself and your injury better than anyone does. That makes you the expert on your needs. We all know overdoing isn't the same as it used to be. Be sure to be kind to yourself.

It is important to trust that it will all work out. As stressful as moving is, people do it every day, and in every walk of life. They all get through it. Some do it with the finesse and style that irritates the rest of us. Some struggle and swear and fight. In the end, the task is still complete no matter the journey. You will get moved, you will learn to be flexible, you will learn just how many things you actually have and don't need, and you will eventually be settled into your new home.

## Meet Tobie-Lynn Andrade

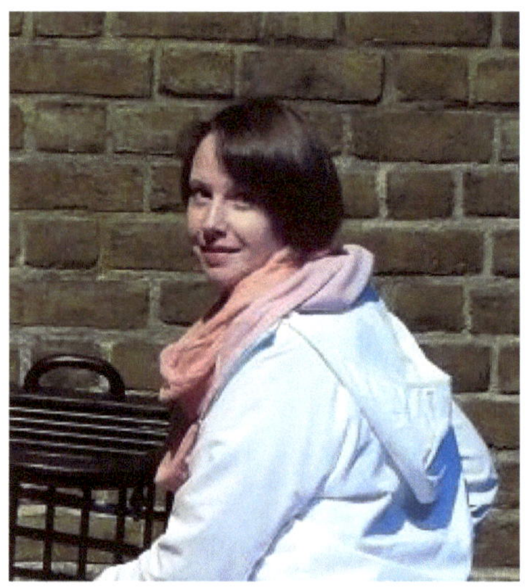

*Tobie-Lynn is a lifelong fan of reading and an avid crafter, as well as a huge Harry Potter geek. She is recovering from a grade three concussion with front left lobe damage and post-concussion syndrome with seizures.*

*Tobie-Lynn is using natural medicines and methods to heal from her injuries, and the Harry Potter stories to help herself heal. One of her greatest moments in life was going to England where the Harry Potter series was filmed and standing with her husband on the actual bridge used in the films.*

# Join our Facebook Family

What do over 25,000 people from over 40 countries and five continents all have in common? They are all members of our vibrant Facebook family at 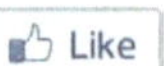/TBIHopeandInspiration

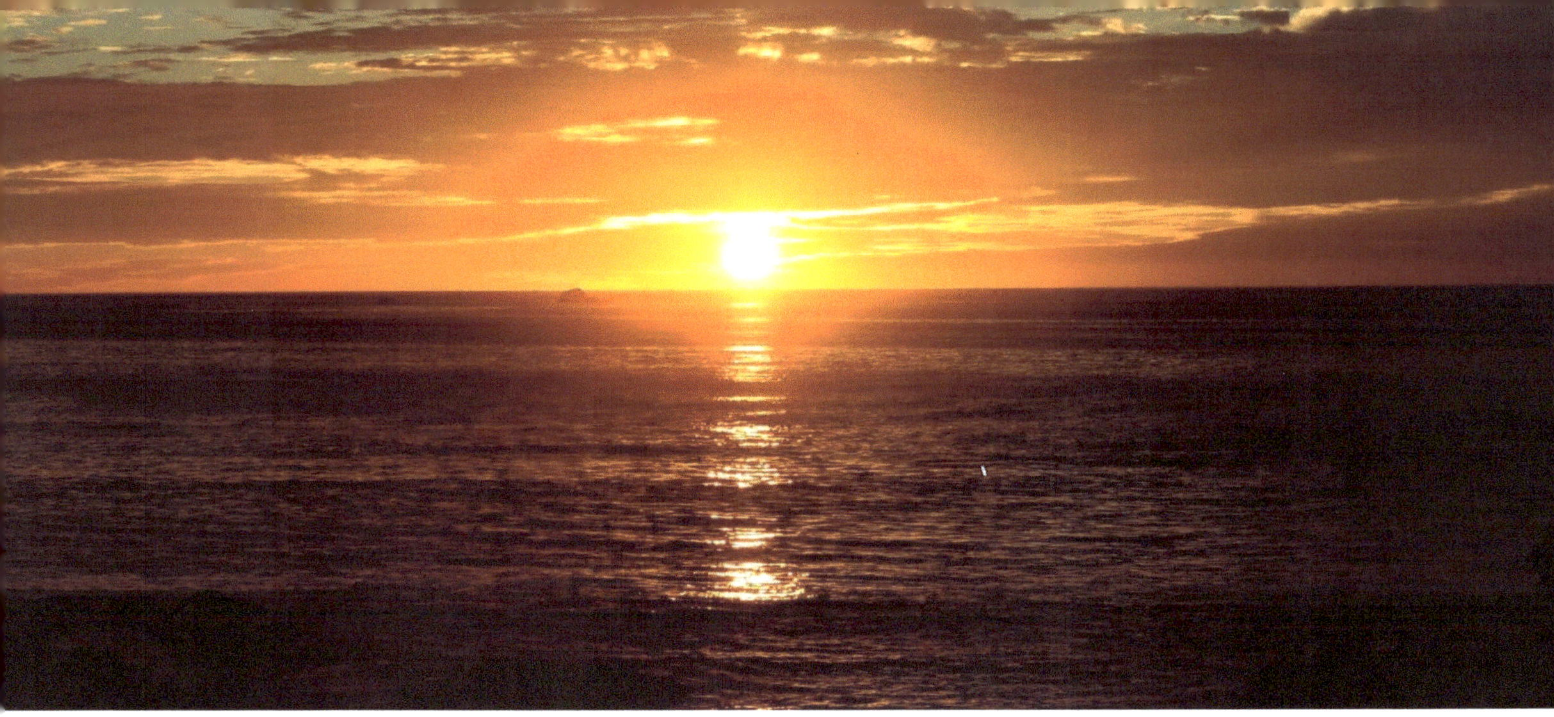

# One More Day

## By Rosemary Rawlins

Recovery is a process. Healing is a process, and some might say we go through life in a constant state of healing from discomforts large and small that our bodies suffer daily. And then there are the big health events — the events that change nearly everything and rearrange our lives in ways we never saw coming.

When my husband, Hugh, sustained a severe traumatic brain injury, my life sped up. I rushed into emergency management mode. I ran to the hospital. I quickly called friends and relatives. Even my heart raced.

And then, just as suddenly, life slowed down to the quiet business of healing — to the steady tick of a slow clock counting down the seconds. While I was waiting in this limbo as I watched my husband heal, my thoughts turned inward. Questions rose up. *What just happened? What does this change mean? Can I handle this?* And the one question many TBI spouses ask themselves: *Will my husband ever be the same? Will I ever be the same?*

The answer I always whispered to myself was, *yes, of course, he'll be the same.* My silent wish was wrong.

The experience of nearly losing Hugh never feels distant or vague, and he is fourteen years out of his accident. The shock of it always feels fresh to me.

When I visit a rehab hospital to speak to therapists or the community, my heart races again. The fluorescent lights and the "clean" smell can propel me back to the spring of 2002 so completely that I have to inhale deeply to calm myself.

When I step in front of a group of TBI families, I see weary faces at the beginning of the healing process, and I want to deliver a huge serving of hope on a shiny platter to them. I want to tell them all will be well, but I can't. All I can honestly tell them is: if your loved one survived, you will need to be patient.

Every brain injury is different, and every recovery is different. There are better treatments and more knowledge about brain injuries than were available fourteen years ago.

There is hope, tempered hope. And there are many people now trying to find a better way to treat brain injuries, but there are no cures and no magic remedies to make your life go back to what it once was.

This is not the best news. And yet, from the podium, I see heads nodding in agreement. I see eyes well up with tears. I see yearning and sorrow, understanding, compassion, and gratitude.

**Every brain injury is different, and every recovery is different. There are better treatments and more knowledge about brain injuries than were available fourteen years ago.**

Somehow, my being honest often comforts families, and that means the world to me. Speaking openly about my struggle, Hugh's struggle and our family's daunting uphill climb gives caregivers and survivors a form of validation that sounds something like this:

*What I am going through is hard; it's very hard.*
*I'm not alone in this aching disconnected experience.*
*I'm not weak. This injury is all encompassing — my problems sometimes feel insurmountable.*
*There are people who understand and can help me.*
*I will eventually be able to make progress and find peace and joy again.*

Sometimes we just need a good friend to sit with as we wait out a stretch of time that seems unending. We just need someone to say, "You will survive this. You can do this one more day." And several years later, you could *be* that someone for someone else.

*Reprinted with permission from BrainLine.org, a WETA website. [www.BrainLine.org](www.BrainLine.org).*

## Meet Rosemary Rawlins

*Rosemary Rawlins is the author of "Learning by Accident: A Caregiver's True Story of Fear, Family, and Hope," an inspirational memoir about learning and growing through adversity.*

*She lives with her family in Glen Allen, VA and Nags Head, NC. She loves to read, write, walk on the beach, laugh out loud, eat chocolate, drink red wine, and spend time with her family and friends.*

*You can learn more about Rosemary at: www.rosemaryrawlins.com*

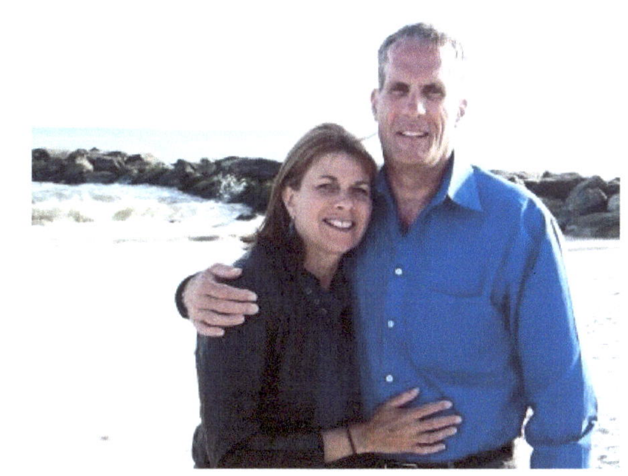

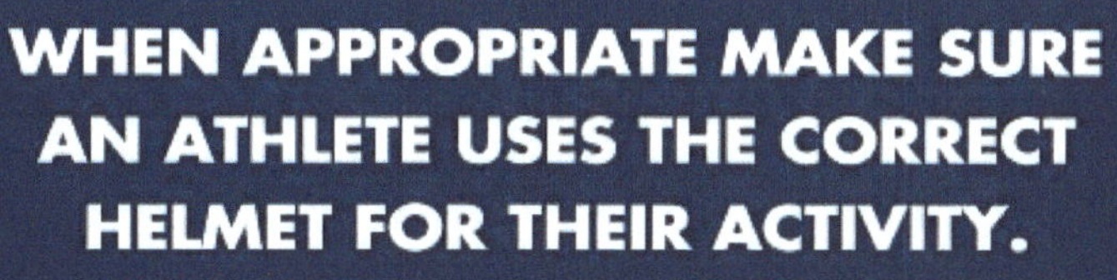


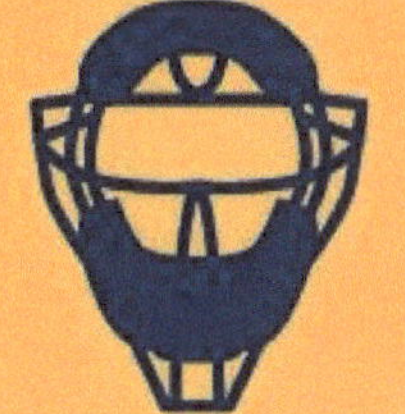

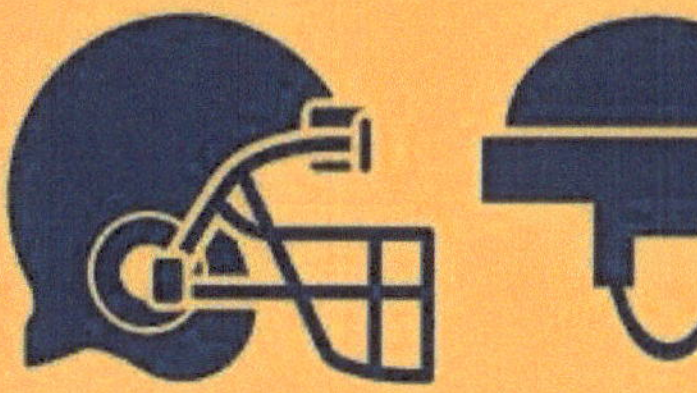

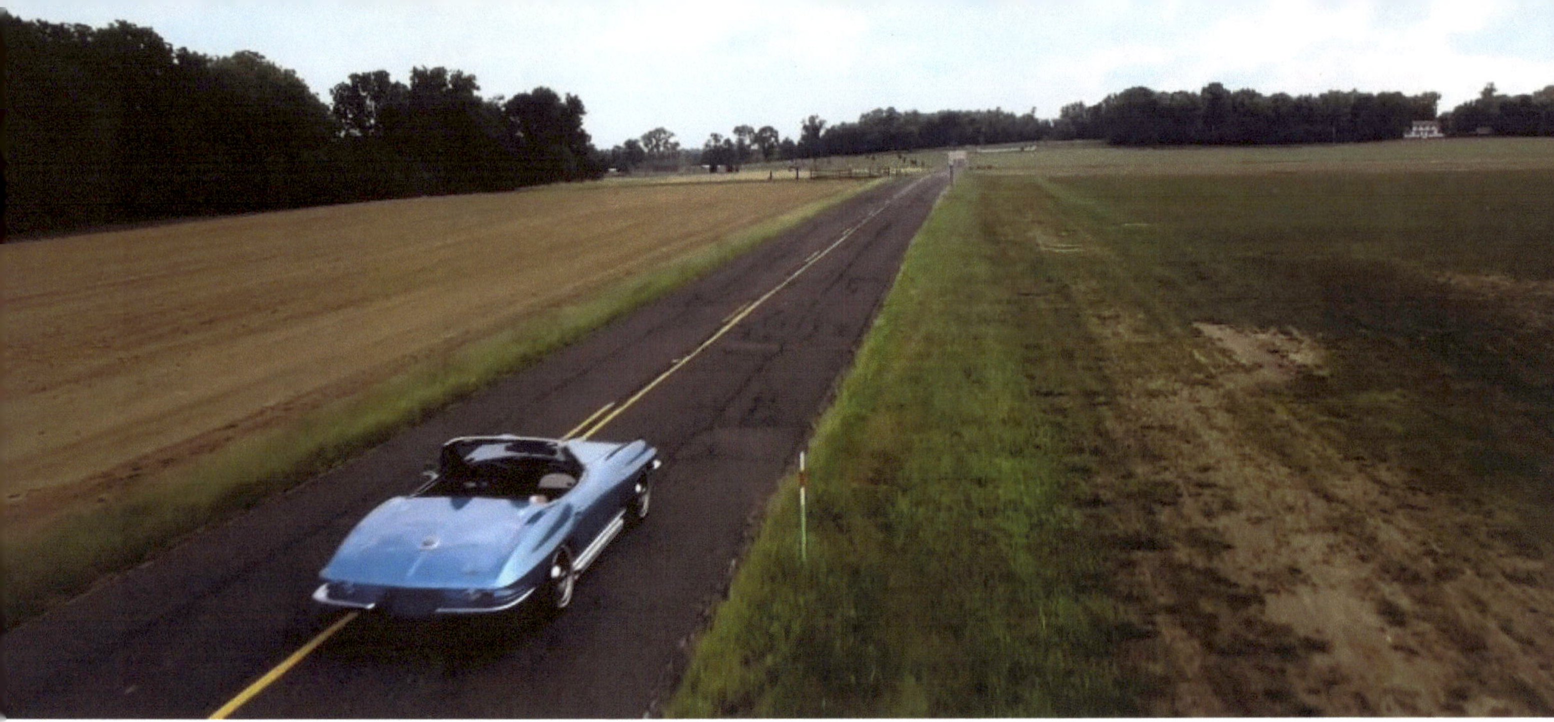

# Moving Forward

## By Ric Johnson

We all know that familiar phrase, "One step forward, and two steps back." Many times that is how I, along with many other survivors, feel. We heard that recovery is a one- or two-year process. We hear that we will plateau. We are told that what we gained back is all we will ever have. We never had to ask for help before the injury that forever changed our lives. Now we are living a life we never planned for or expected. For too many, that is when despair starts to set in.

For me, today is pretty much the same as yesterday. Tomorrow will probably be nearly the same as today, depending on whether or not I have an appointment to attend. I cannot really complain about my "current" normal. When I feel like I am moving sideways, what can I do to keep moving forward? How do I make today better than yesterday? How do I add new items into my recovery toolbox?

> "I do like regular daily tasks, but regular day-to-day processes should not guide my day."

I do like regular daily tasks, but regular day-to-day processes should not guide my day. Moving forward is really about changing directions. Step 1 has to be getting to the bathroom (of course), but why is drinking my first cup of coffee always my second step? How about getting dressed before walking to the kitchen? Why not make the bed, then get dressed, then drink a cup of coffee? There are many steps taken during a day, steps that I can control. Control means I have to put on my thinking cap. My injury and my PTSD have to become second fiddle.

Things like worries about falling, worries about aphasia, worries about short-term memory, and worrying about nearly everything keep me moving sideways. In fact, worry moves me back to my first year or two.

After over fourteen years, I have learned how to react to situations I was not expecting. Do I react as I always do? If yes, why? Wasn't a different step available? Maybe I did not have time to find that other step. Maybe, maybe, maybe.

"Maybe" is almost my curse. I need to be heading for the light. My post-injury life is not a tunnel, so the light I need to head into is the moving forward light. To believe in myself, to know that I did all I could do yesterday, a week ago, or a month ago means I should be able to do it today. Just think before starting. Moving forward is a big gain, even when doing a simple repeatable task.

Maybe watching TV, listening to talk-radio stations, or calling friends just to pass the time does not seem like a "problem," but my brain needs to exercise to continue to rewire itself to keep moving forward.

What kind of exercises? Playing a card game, taking a walk outside, having lunch in the backyard, opening a window and listening to the sounds of my neighborhood.

Is there a task to do that I have been procrastinating? Yep, I should have worked on that one a year ago however, I let it go every day. I have to make that a top priority to start and finish.

Instead of calling any day my "new" normal, I have now renamed it as my "current" normal. Why? Because my recovery has not stopped and is going well. During the first couple of years, everything was brand new. Now, after fourteen years, things are not new, just different. I am always surprised when what didn't work a week ago, is now fine, or at least better. I believe that happens because I am still recovering.

First, and maybe the best part of my recovery, is to continue going to support group meetings. Talking with other survivors and hearing their tips and techniques. Those survivors are also able to ask us to share our tips or techniques. Sure, not everyone is able to use every trick. Even if what I am trying to use does not fix my needs, it will probably give me a new process to think about and add to my toolbox.

Perhaps the most important thing about my monthly support group meetings is my ability to help other survivors with their recovery. In fact, I am not writing this article all by myself. It is being written by other members of my support group as well. How? By writing down all the information during our meetings. Because of a limited short-term memory, I have to write notes to myself.  Without notes, I know I will forget.

The second piece of my recovery is to make myself aware of myself, which helps me to get out of being stuck in a loop. Recovery is an amazing part of living, but it needs us to rename our new normal as our current normal. Like life itself, this will change over time, but that is one of the key aspects to brain injury recovery – learning to adapt and change.


## Meet Ric Johnson

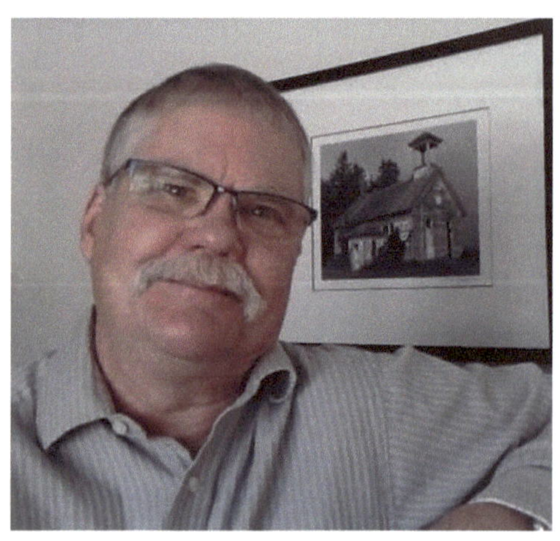

*Ric Johnson is a husband, father, grandfather, and a traumatic brain injury survivor from just over fourteen years.*

*Ric is also a member of the Speaker Bureau for the Minnesota Brain Injury Alliance, and facilitator for The Courage Kenny Brain Injury Support Group.*

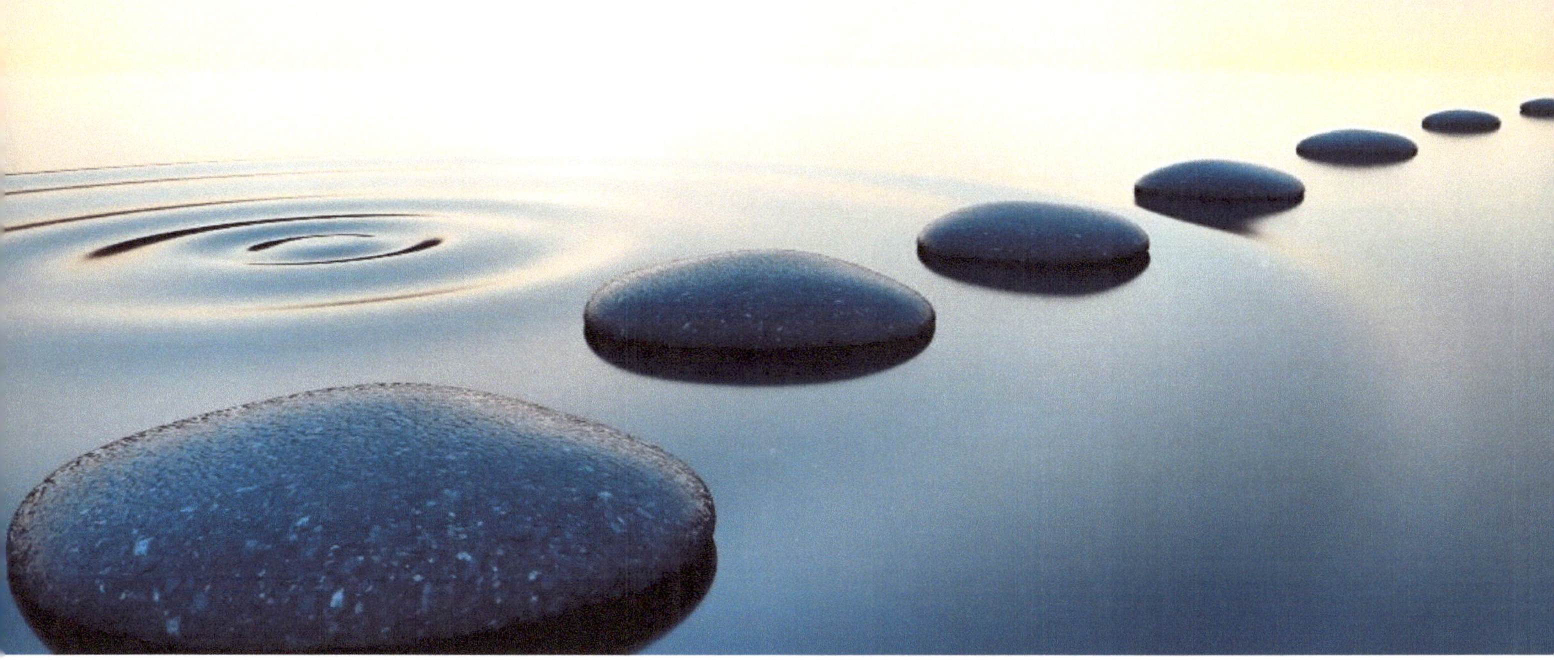

# Changing Roles

**By Christine Lawrence**

"Happy to help!" "The feelings you are experiencing are normal and you will get through this." "I will see you next week for our session." I said these words many times while I was still a professional therapist. However, these words have a different meaning now that the therapist is the patient.

I experienced my Traumatic Brain Injury after a car accident in 2016, when I was hit by a Mack truck. The expression, "I felt like I was hit by a Mack truck," which I said thousands of times prior to the accident, took on a whole new meaning. I hear that expression used today and I chuckle and say, "you have no idea what that really feels like!"

> "As a professional therapist, however, I was used to providing care for others personally and professionally."

I can laugh at this now. As a professional therapist, however, I was used to providing care for others personally and professionally. I was the fixer and the problem solver. Control played a huge part in those actions.

As a TBI survivor, my struggle to let go of the control was not just physical, but it was emotional, mental, and spiritual. I was not in control of my brain functions, as I wanted my brain to work a certain way. I was angry, confused, hurt, depressed and disappointed that it had failed me. The control I thought I once had was not there and I did not like it.

My therapy included rehabilitation, physical, ocular, speech, occupational and counseling. Throughout my intake sessions with each professional, I remember crying through the questions and yet still being in disbelief that I was not sitting in the big chair, asking the questions.

**Receiving help is not a sign of weakness.**

Receiving help is a sign of recognizing that healing needs to take place with the help of others and the community.

**Resiliency is our strength**.

A wise neuro psychologist said, the only way out is through one of our sessions. I was trying to avoid the internal pain and that when your world turns upside-down, it is not fun.

However, each session we attend, each medication we take for the pain, each counseling session we mourn and cry and get up and do it again the next day, we are putting our strength in action and forging a new path.

**Mind and body connection is a real thing**.

When I started to journal, do yoga, or seek nature, I felt a small window in my soul open. A different part of my brain was activated in spite of my cognitive difficulties – a different part started to sing. Do you ever wonder why people do not stutter when they sing but stutter when they talk?

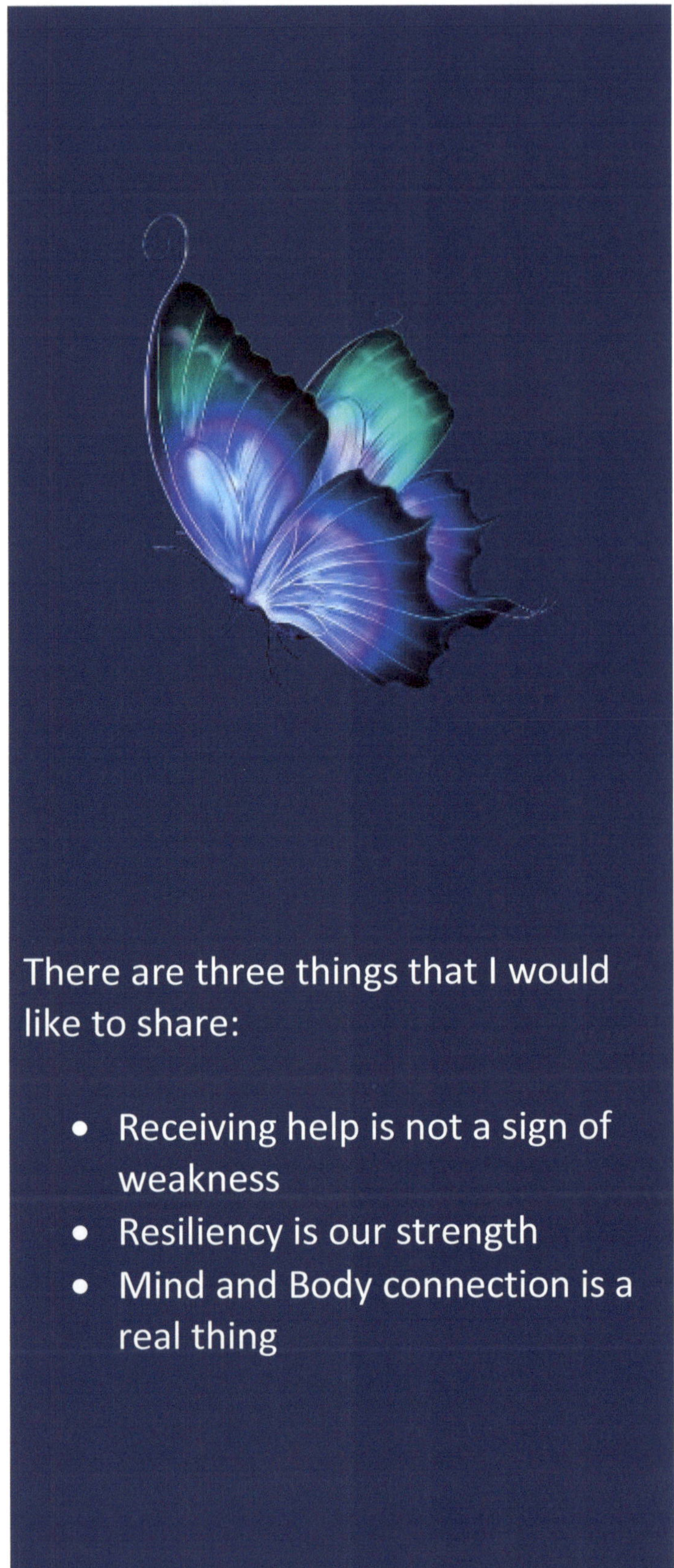

When I started singing/chanting, and noticed that I sounded pretty clear, I understood a different part of my brain was working.

As a TBI survivor, I have days when I need to recall these three things on my list. I share these three things with you to offer encouragement on your healing journey. I might not be able to sit in the "big chair" right now, however, the chair or mat I am sitting on is quite comfortable for learning and listening.

May the light in me recognize the light in you. Namaste.

## Meet Christine Lawrence

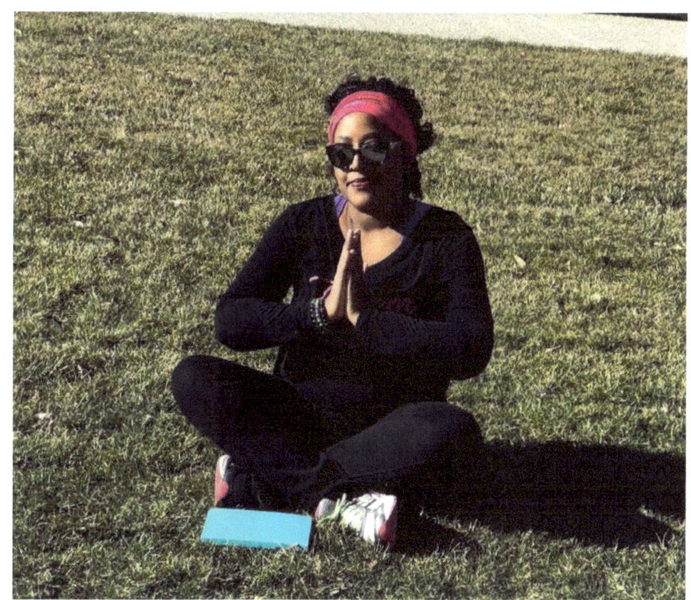

Christine Lawrence is a TBI survivor and Yoga teacher student. After her car accident in 2016, Christine was initiated into the TBI world.

Christine's career included counseling, program development/director. Christine now hopes to incorporate advocacy - for the TBI world open to career paths.

She continues to rebuild and learn her new brain. She hopes to assist others in the healing journey and assist with trauma work, as she continues to heal.

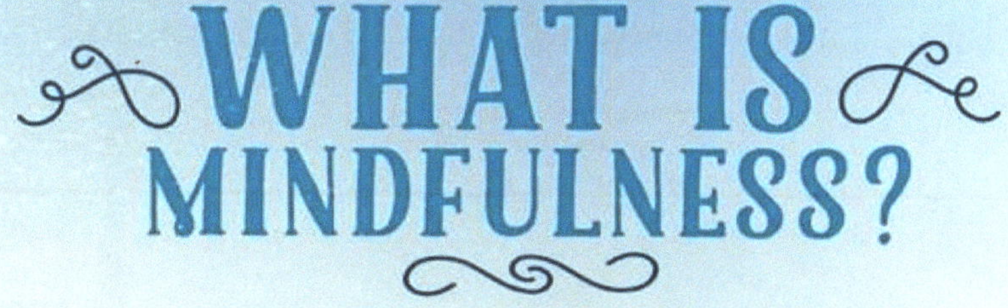

# INTRODUCING THE NEW
# dish FLEX PACK
## Create Your Own TV Package

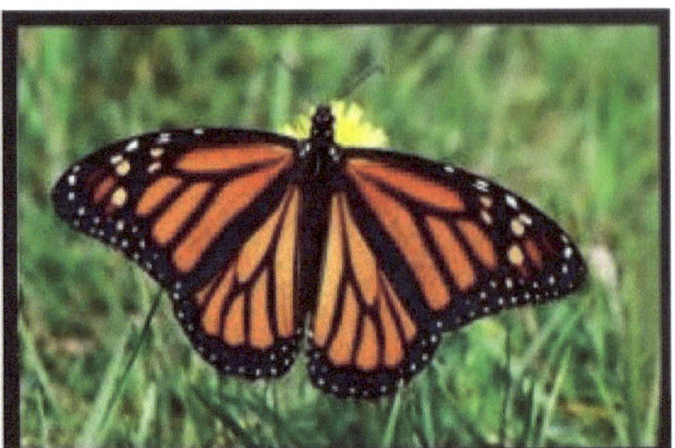

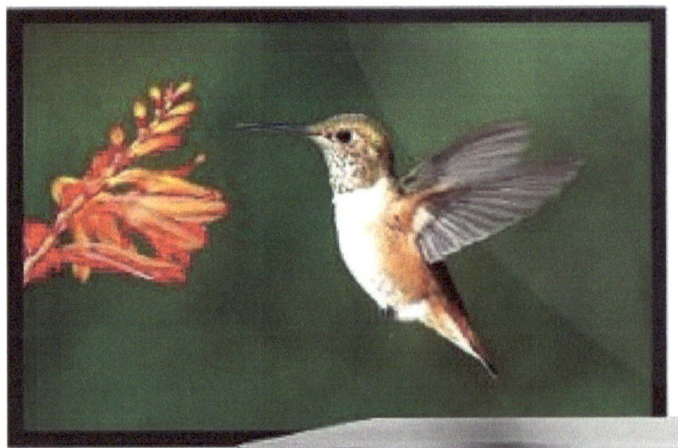

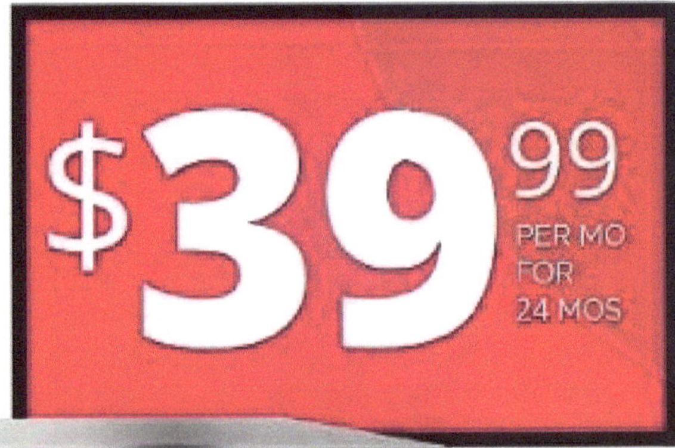


**Free Streaming**

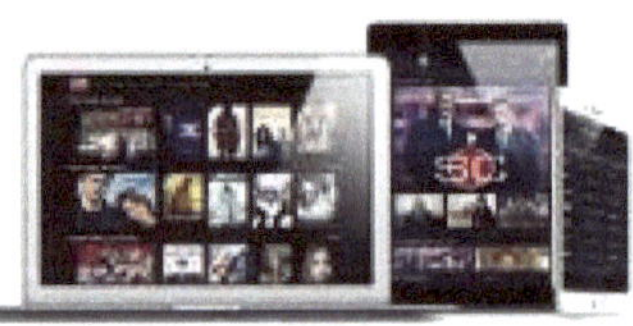


+

**Free Installation**

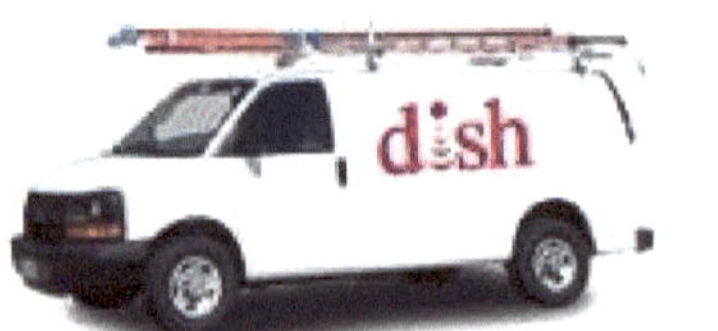

+

**Add Internet**

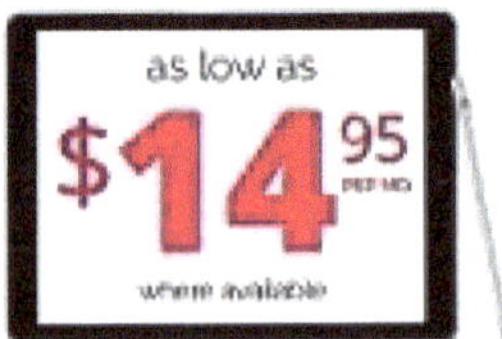


## Call 1-800-391-1328

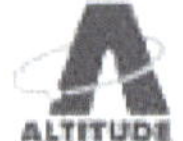

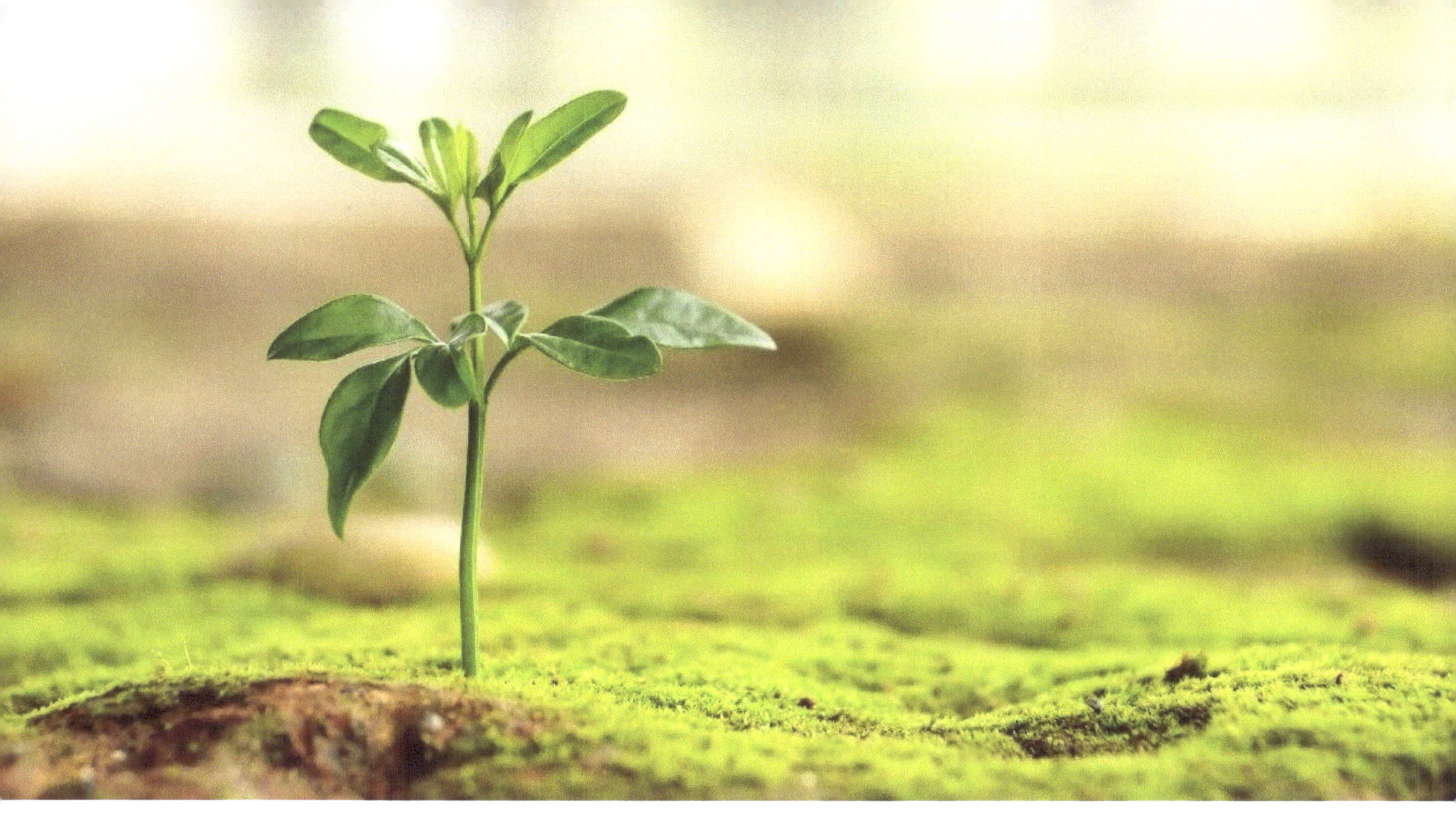

# The Many Faces of Brain Injury and Grief

## By Norma Myers

Our journey, one chosen for us, not by us, has been described as complex, unthinkable, unimaginable. It is all those descriptions and so many more.

What started out as brothers spending a Sunday together, ended in tragedy when Aaron's truck unexplainably hit a tree. The same fatal impact causing Aaron's death and Steven's Traumatic Brain Injury (TBI), caused irreversible heart damage to their parents, the kind of damage that is incurable. We are told time will help, but more than five years have passed, and the pain doesn't subside. We just learn to live with and tolerate it.

> "We are told time will help, but more than five years have passed, and the pain doesn't subside."

Throughout my life, I have held many titles, but none as prestigious as wife to my husband Carlan and mom to our two sons. I never imagined

I would add the titles of survivor and caregiver to my portfolio on the same day. All at once, I was a survivor for surviving the death of my first-born son, Aaron, and a caregiver for my son, Steven, who sustained a TBI. Being thrust into the foreign world of caregiving, coupled with grieving the earthly separation from Aaron, left my body physically depleted and consumed with shock, a kind of shock that numbed me.

The numbness allowed me to function but prevented me from clearly seeing the ocean of faces affected by Steven's TBI and Aaron's death. As the shock began to fade, it felt like a curtain lifted, and I was cast in a play with all the characters, one by one revealing how they were affected.

Amidst their grief, they wondered if I would ever laugh again, have date nights or travel. They wondered how this trauma would affect my marriage and my friendships. Their fears, mingled with those of our own, weighed on our minds. After all, how can you think about experiencing happiness when your world has been turned upside down by a diagnosis, with an integral part of your family suddenly gone?

The face of grief that makes my heart skip a beat daily is that of Steven. As if life with a TBI isn't challenging enough, despite his pain, he bravely faces each day without his brother, his best friend. As Mom, I want to fix it, but I can't. I can only remind him that Aaron would expect us to make the most of each day, even when we don't think we can.

I hope my words convey the message that while it took time to regain our equilibrium, we sincerely acknowledge *your* loss and pain.



I hope my words convey the message that while it took time to regain our equilibrium, we sincerely acknowledge *your* loss and pain.

There are no adequate words to express our gratitude for the role you played in making a difference in Steven's recovery while putting your pain on hold to provide strength to me and my family in our time of desperate need.

Some examples of the Many Faces of TBI and Grief:

- Good Samaritans that found our sons and stayed until help arrived.
- Fire and rescue team ensuring our sons made it safely off the mountain.
- The trauma team that embraced the magnitude of our loss, refusing to give up on saving Steven's life.
- Family and friends that kept vigil by our side at the hospital as Steven fought for his life, and stood by us as we celebrated Aaron's life. You stayed, seamlessly switching gears working behind the scenes, taking care of everything that we could not.
- Aaron and Steven's friends that showed up at the hospital and funeral, not knowing what to say. They did the most important thing; they showed up.
- Expected Moms in the visitation line with tears streaming down their faces, those tears an acknowledgment of my pain.
- Co-workers from employers past and present, eagerly showing their support.
- Our community on standby to come to our rescue, and without fail they did.
- Healthcare providers. Many have stayed the course, proudly witnessing Steven's miraculous recovery.

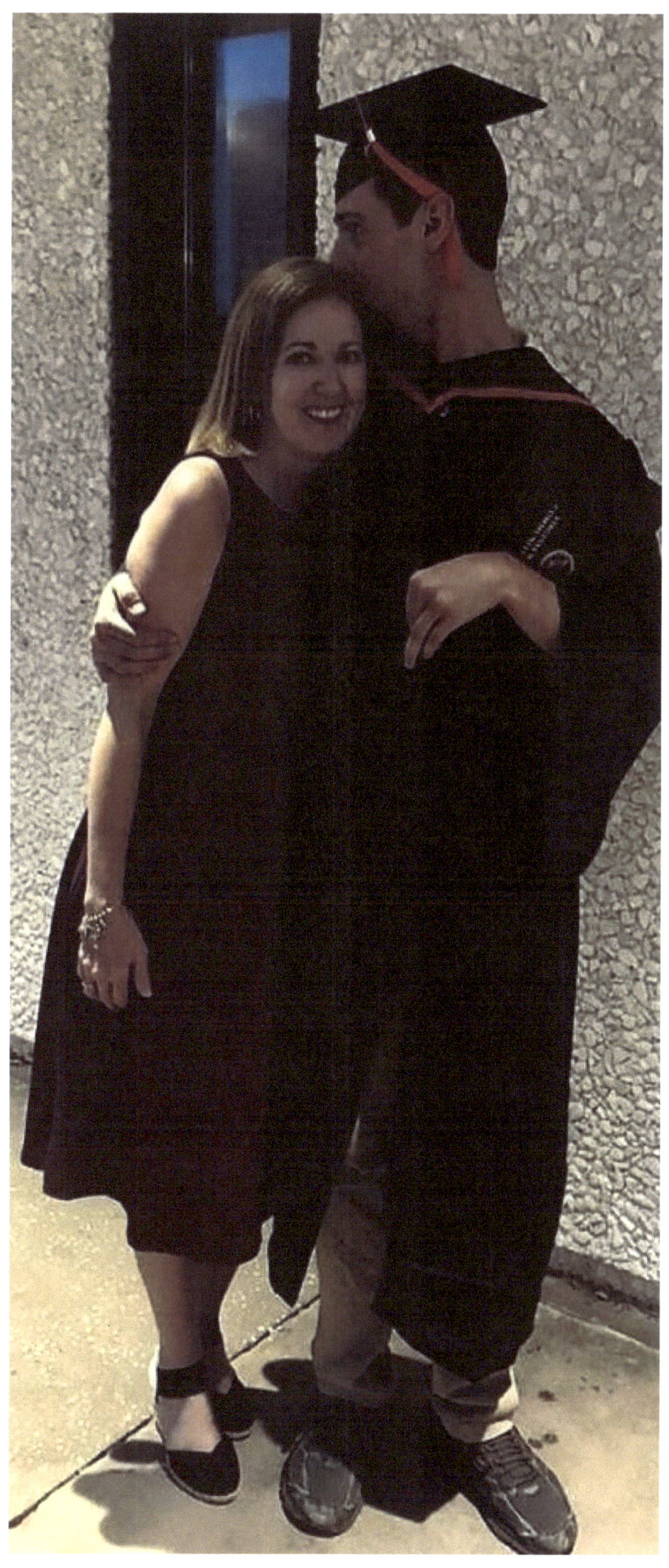

- Charity foundations that said, "Yes," we will help.
- Our TBI Community—near and far—offering support and resources.
- Steven's Trauma team that encouraged us to reach out to other family members facing loss.

We have experienced the double-sided emotions of birthdays, holidays and anniversaries, a time when happiness collides with grief as we simultaneously celebrate Steven's recovery and Aaron's death.

A dear friend recently shared her thoughts on two very *impactful* words: **acknowledge** and **accept**. These words deeply struck a chord in my heart. I **can** acknowledge and accept Steven's TBI, after all, he's here! While I acknowledge Aaron's death, my heart **will not** and **cannot** accept losing a son at the tender age of 26, with his life ahead of him. No parent should have to live with this unnatural pain.

I believe that God brings those that we need into our lives at just the right moment, for such crucial times as **then** and **now**. Some of the faces affected by our journey showed up on day one, others, year one, and now almost five years later, are still showing up, right on time. It takes a village. We're forever thankful that you are an integral part of ours.

**Meet Norma Myers**

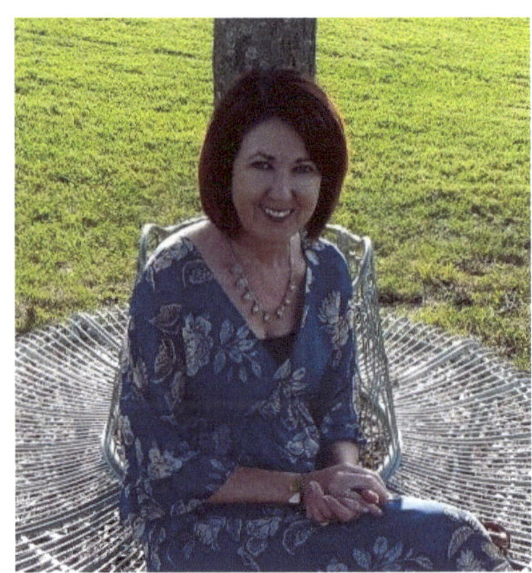

*Norma and her husband Carlan spend much of their time supporting their son Steven as he continues on his road to recovery. Norma is an advocate for those recovering from traumatic brain injury.*

*Her written work has been featured on Brainline.org, a multi-media website that serves the brain injury community. Her family continues to heal.*

# In prosperity, our friends know us; in adversity, we know our friends.

~John Churton Collins

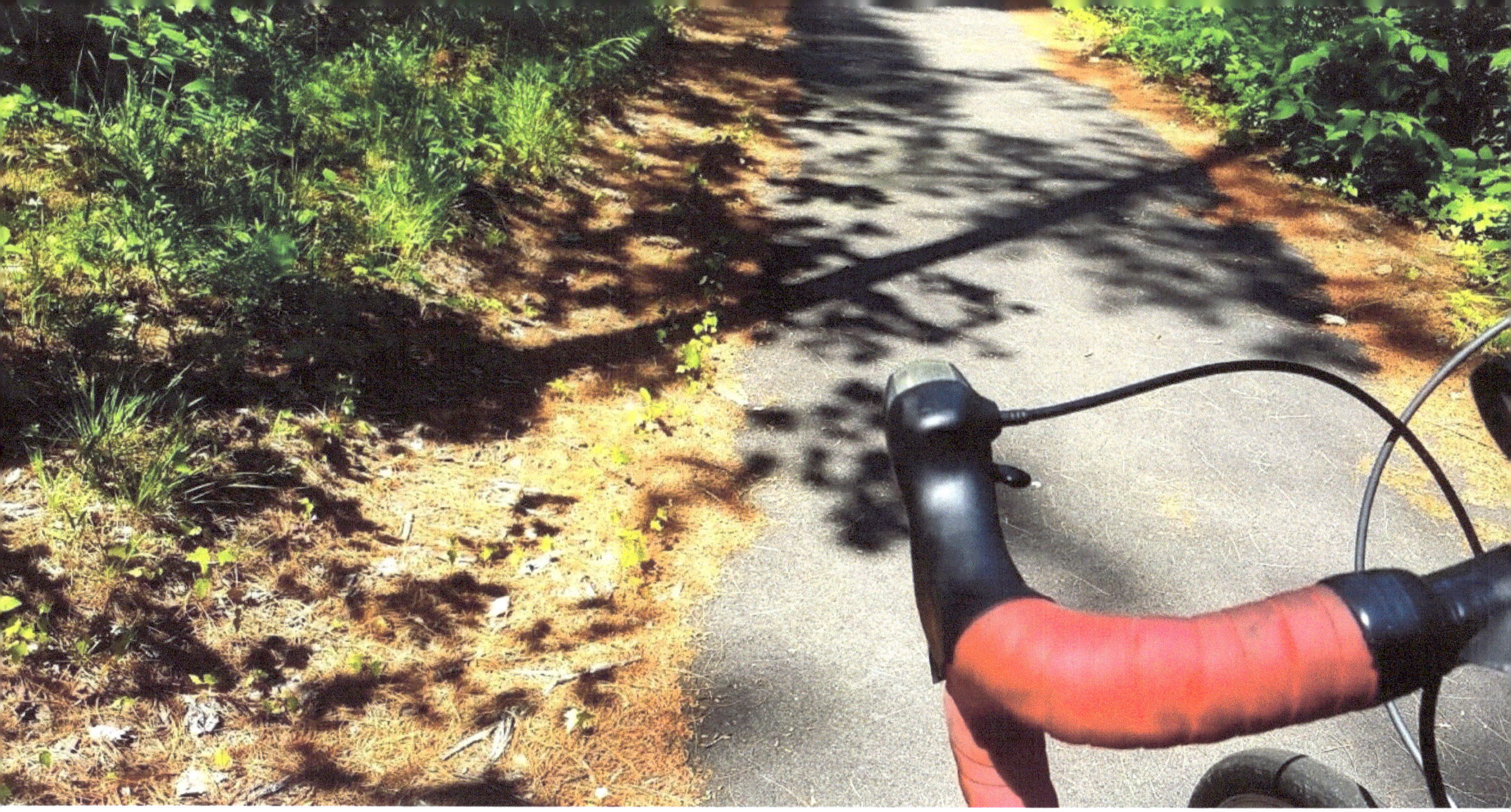

# The Only Normal I Know

**By David A. Grant**

I was recently out for a bike ride. It's been seven years after my traumatic brain injury, and I still cycle daily. There are a myriad of reasons. The first one is the most obvious – I love cycling. There is something magical being out on the streets, enjoying a totally immersive experience.

Of course, there are the health benefits. I am diabetic, and daily cardio helps keep my diabetes in check. I get the dubious luxury of snacking a bit without gaining too much weight. In addition, over the last few years, there has been a growing body of evidence that daily cardio speeds brain injury recovery. Mindful of all this, I would be crazy not to cycle.

> "For a few minutes, sadness consumed me as I thought about how things used to be."

During my recent ride, music came on that I listened to the summer before my injury. It was the summer of 2010, my last summer before everything changed. For a few minutes, sadness consumed me as I thought about how things used to be.

I started thinking about "normal."

Shortly after my injury, I heard someone describe life after brain injury as "the new normal." Frankly, I could not stand that phrase.

There was *nothing* normal about my life during those difficult early years after my injury. The very foundation of my personality shifted. Friends dropped out of my life; family members faded to black, and financial stressors kept me as awake at night as my PTSD nightmares did. Life itself had become a veritable nightmare.

People had the audacity to call this my *new normal.* There was nothing even remotely normal about that existence. Sarah and I were struggling daily just to regain our footing. It remains the biggest single event in both of our lives. I steadfastly refused to accept that things were going to be like that for the long haul. The never-ending parade of challenges made life unsustainable.

Ladies and gentlemen, if you are looking for "normal," it's a setting on your dishwasher.

One of the blessings of time is that it passes. For those new to the wacky, unexplainable realm of brain injury, let me share something that I have learned over the years: Time is your friend.

While I never accepted my early post-injury chaos as normal, my life today is pretty— dare I say it—normal. My wife Sarah and I live reasonably uneventful lives, something I say with profound gratitude.

My perception of normal has shifted since my injury. Today it is normal to lose words and have speech challenges when I am overtired or stressed. It is also normal to take more time than I did before my TBI to process simple requests.

> **People had the audacity to call this my *new normal.* There was nothing even remotely normal about that existence.**

It is normal to have my ears never stop ringing. It is normal to have a wave of emotion crash over me that brings me to tears. It is normal to say too much, too candidly. It is also normal to tell the people I am closest to that I love them and that my life is enriched because of their presence.

Sometimes the lack of a filter can be a good thing.

Let's circle back to my recent ride, shall we? As I thought about a normal life, two things came to mind. First, I have trouble really recalling what life was like before my injury. As the years continue to pass, my life before my brain injury is not only forgotten, but somehow seems less important than it did in the early years of my recovery. Second, and probably more importantly, my life today with all its quirks and challenges is really the only normal I know. The volume has been turned down on a few of my more glaring deficits. And those that remain, well, I've learned to live with them.

Over the last few months, I have had quite a few people tell me that I seem happier than I've been in a while. While I have never really been unhappy, feeling that my life is reasonably normal does bring with it a bit of peace. In the end, that's all most of us want - a bit of peace in the midst of this one shot at life.

## Meet David A. Grant

*David A. Grant is a freelance writer based out of southern New Hampshire and the publisher of HOPE Magazine. He is the author of Metamorphosis, Surviving Brain Injury.*

*He is also a contributing author to Chicken Soup for the Soul, Recovering from Traumatic Brain Injuries. David is a BIANH Board Member. David is a regular contributing writer to Brainline.org, a PBS sponsored website.*

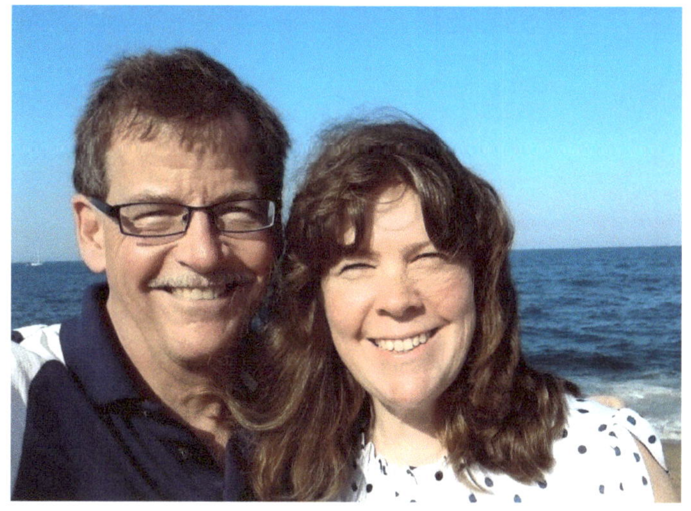

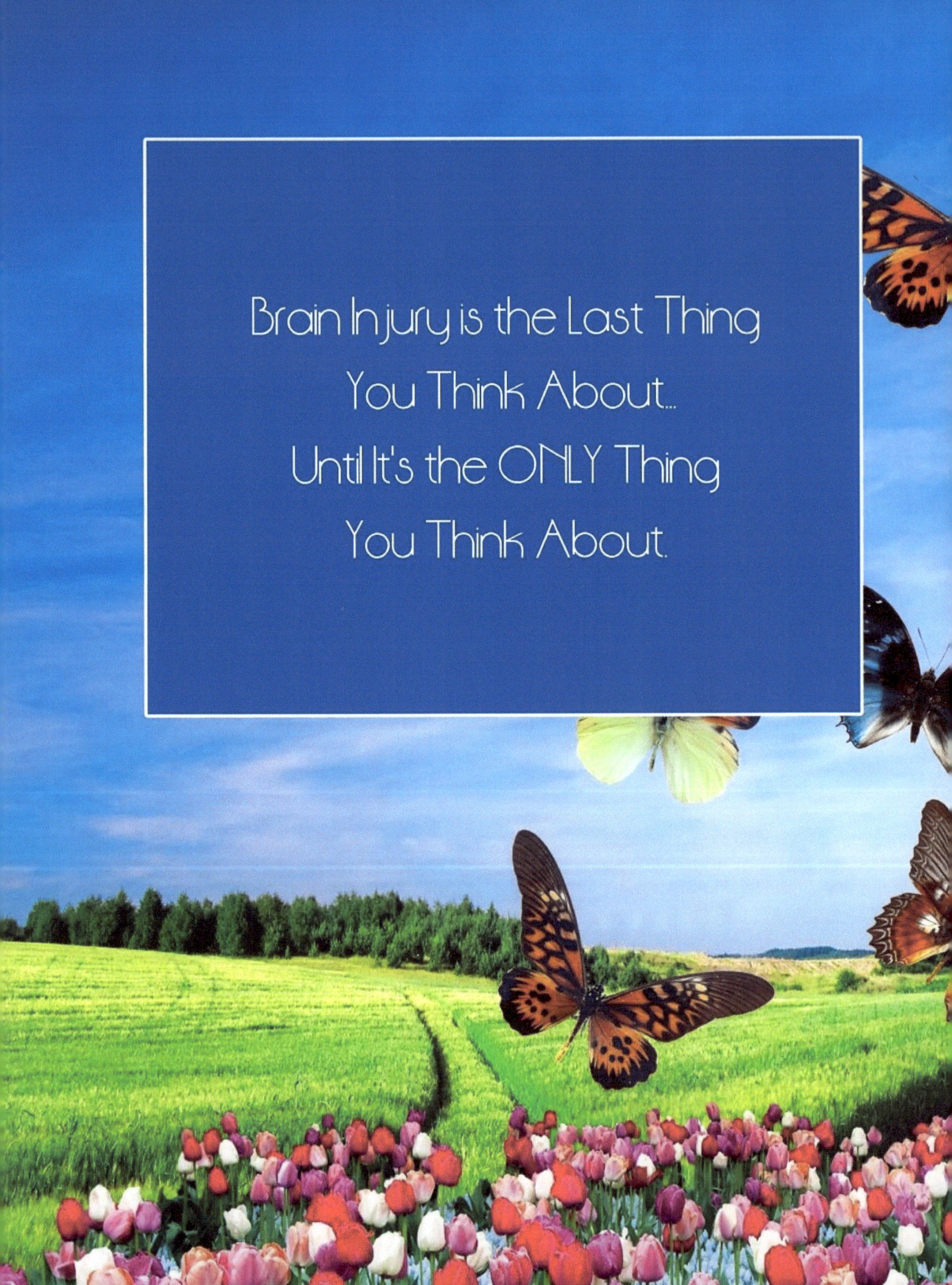

Brain Injury is the Last Thing
You Think About...
Until It's the ONLY Thing
You Think About.

# Grasp The Life Ring

## By Donavan Vliet

In a moment's notice
Traumatic brain injury strikes
It catches you when you are least aware
It arrives unannounced
Scrambling your mind.

Putting the pieces back together
Is like creating a puzzle
It takes time to recreate the image
It may seem you are normal
Nonetheless the hidden disabilities are real.

You may feel unqualified to respond
Yet the new you gives you strength
The urge to move forward
There is no going back to the former self
Wishing the life-changing event never occurred
Doesn't change the outcome of the jolting
incident.

As the fog clears you seek to recover
The new life may be better than the former
Still it can be a struggle
Living up to your potential is practical
There is no correct path in life.

We all lose our way sometimes
Life is what you make of it
Traumatic brain injury need not hold you back
Grasp the life rings others toss you
The journey need not be taken in despair
I'm here to give you care.

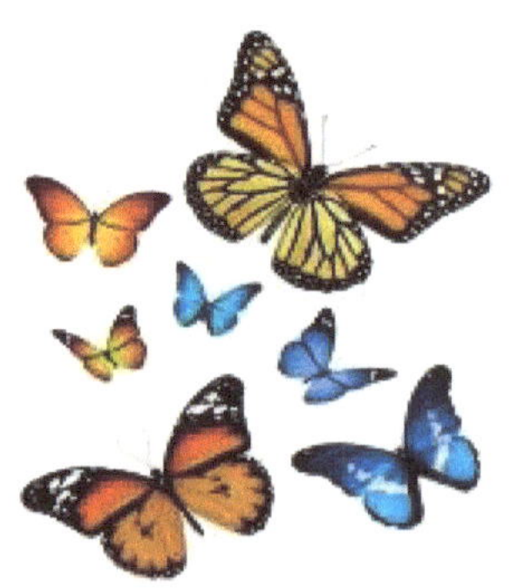

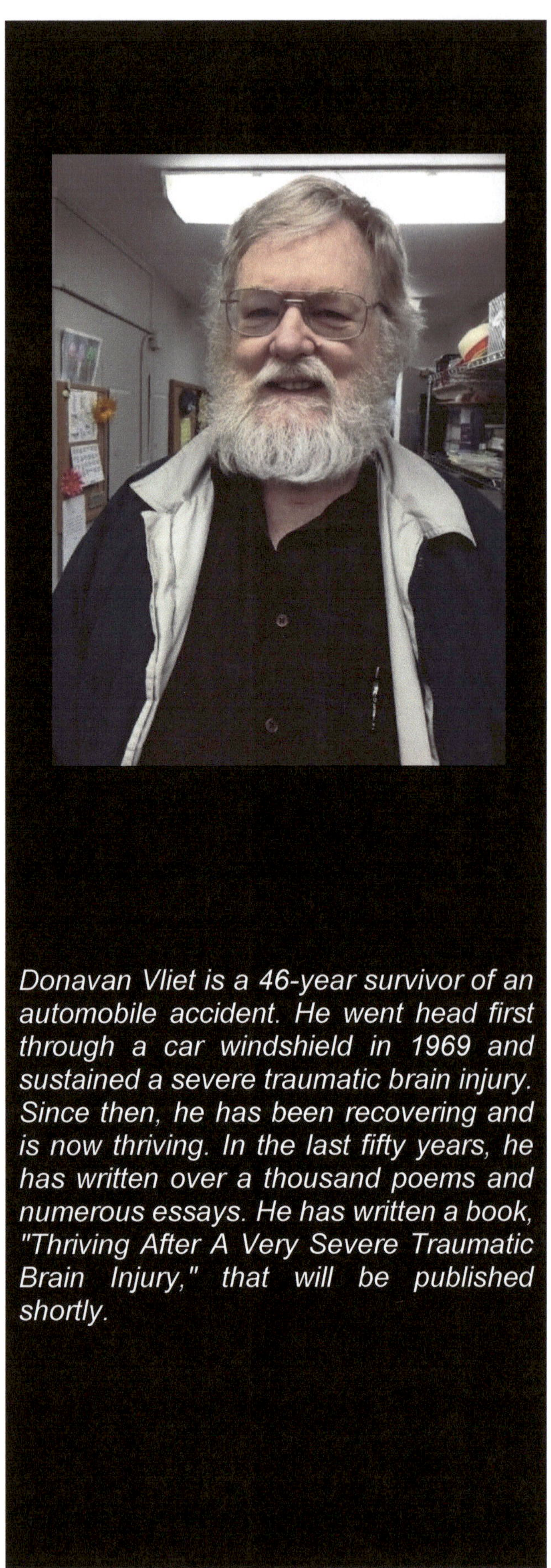

*Donavan Vliet is a 46-year survivor of an automobile accident. He went head first through a car windshield in 1969 and sustained a severe traumatic brain injury. Since then, he has been recovering and is now thriving. In the last fifty years, he has written over a thousand poems and numerous essays. He has written a book, "Thriving After A Very Severe Traumatic Brain Injury," that will be published shortly.*

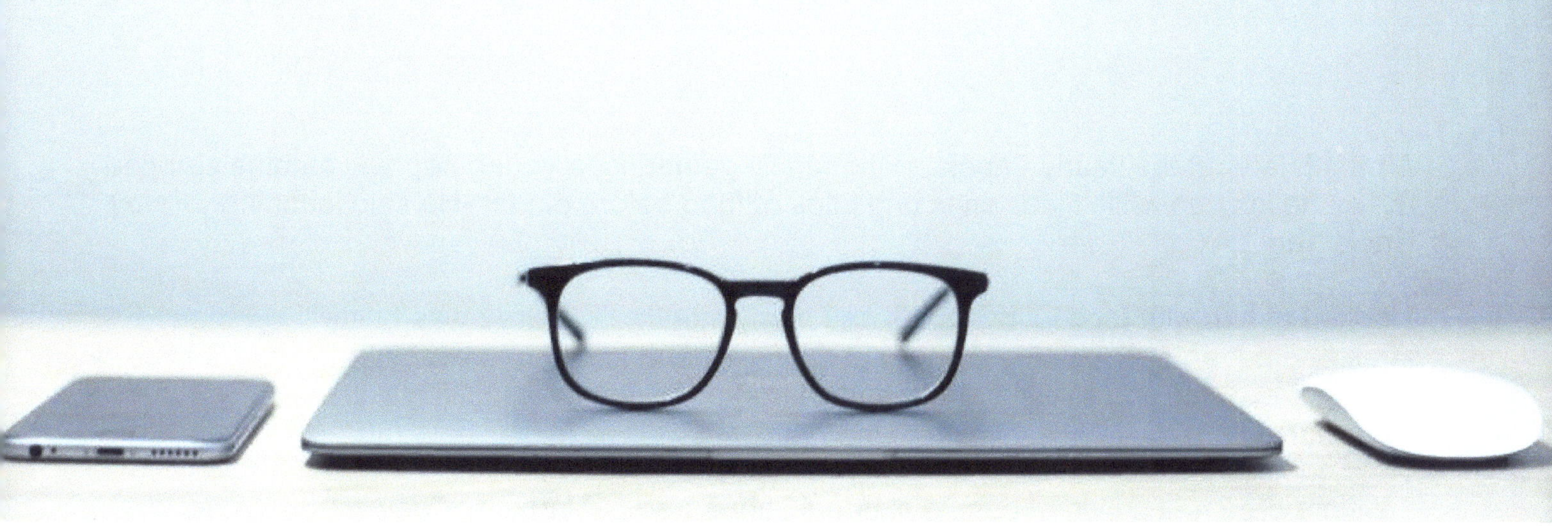

# Overlooked Vision Problems
**By Ted Stachulski**

On a very windy, fall New England day, the engine of the truck I was driving overheated. I pulled off into the breakdown lane of the very busy interstate highway I was traveling so I could see what was happening under the hood. As vehicles sped by well over the speed limit, I opened the heavy, metal hood and propped it up with the metal rod that was designed to hold it up. I then leaned over the front of the truck and saw a coolant hose had become disconnected. That was an easy fix for me because I had a screwdriver I could use to tighten the clamp after I reconnected the hose.

In a split second, a very strong gust of wind blew the hood back to the windshield. The metal rod that had once propped it up fell and hit me on the nose. The wind then quickly reversed direction and slammed the heavy steel hood down onto the top, front, right side of my head. The hard blow, which I would equate to a Professional Wrestler jumping off the top rope to slam his opponent on the head with an 80-pound solid steel chair, knocked me out. I fell backward from a standing position and hit the back of my head on the hard pavement behind me.

> "The wind then quickly reversed direction and slammed the heavy steel hood down onto the top, front, right side of my head."

It ended up being the worst brain injury I'd ever had. An emergency department doctor told me I had a concussion and that I would be good to go back to work in a few days. Having racked up many concussions playing youth sports, I knew he was wrong and that this brain injury was different from all the rest.

A month later at the yearly Thanksgiving family gathering, a young nephew of mine stopped me in the kitchen while I was sneaking bites of food before dinner. He said laughingly, "Hey, Uncle Ted!"

I looked at him with food in my hands and in my mouth. For sure I was busted! He then stretched out an arm, pointed a finger at my face,  and asked in amazement, "How is *that eye* (my right eye) looking straight at me and *that eye* (my left eye) looking at the clock on the wall over there?"

Like in a dream, a crowd of people suddenly appeared behind him. They were looking, squinting, peering and pointing at my face trying to see what my nephew had noticed. As soon as they saw the discrepancy with my eyes, they began laughing at me like I was a sideshow exhibit.

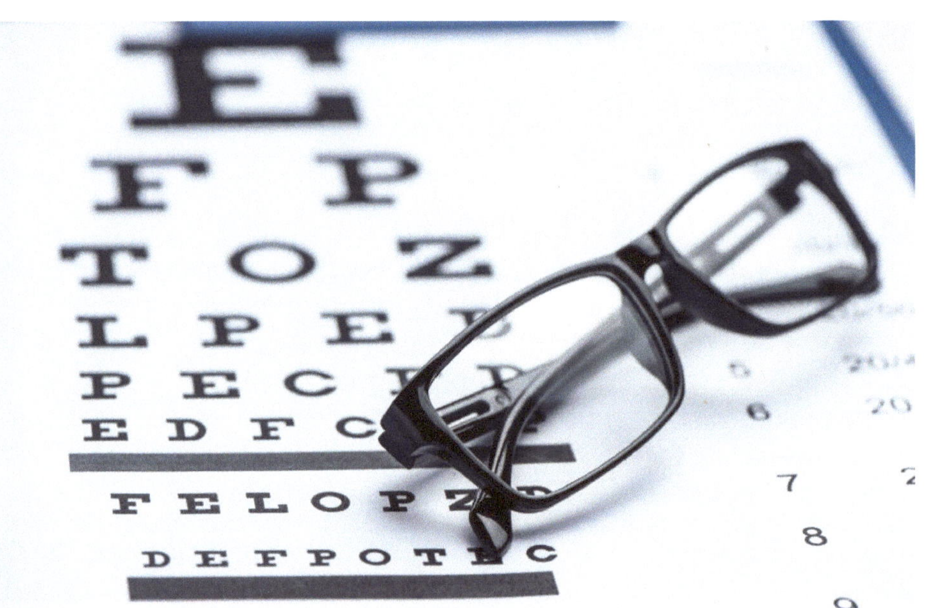

I stood there like a deer in headlights, still suffering from post-concussion symptoms and thought to myself, "This is not good!"

The dream I thought I was in was now turning into a nightmare!

A few days later, I had an appointment with a local Ophthalmologist. He did a quick eye exam and told me I had third and fourth Cranial Nerve Palsy. This is damage to nerves that control eye muscle movements. My left eye was turned outward and upward. He advised me, "This sometimes corrects itself and may take up to a year to do so." I did not really have a lot of visual symptoms and the eye doctor said my brain was, "compensating for the misalignment."

So when I walked out of his office without any solutions on how to improve my vision such as special lenses or vision therapy, I hoped for the best and that my brain would fix itself. Over the next 12 months, however, my nightmare turned into a full-blown horror movie!

Everything in my life that was once enjoyable became extremely stressful for me. I became easily over-stimulated because my brain's filters no longer worked properly. I became overwhelmed by what I saw, heard, touched, or smelled. The persistent, nerve-rattling anxiety prevented me from shopping in a grocery store, sitting in a movie theater, walking around a mall, attending my children's school functions and sporting events, working as an electro-mechanical assembler or driving my car.

At work, detailed electronic schematics and mechanical drawings became too overwhelming to look at. Words jumped all over the page when I tried to read technical manuals. I could not see in 3D anymore and became stuck in a 2D world. I could not imagine and turn images in my brain like I once was able to do and it killed my creativity. My hand-eye coordination was completely off. I dropped expensive parts on the floor because I misjudged where the table I was placing them on was located. I walked into stationary objects because my vision dragged as I turned my head or walked around. All of this led to me making many mistakes and falling behind on required production.

I walked from my workstation to get something at the other end of the shop. As I stood there confused as to what I was down there for, the owner of the company (who had been secretly watching me) stepped out from behind a cabinet and asked, "Ted, why are you down here?"

My eyes filled up with tears as I stood there horrified not knowing what I was looking for. I somberly replied, "I don't know."

He said to me with a very concerned look on his face and tone of voice, "You'd better go get some help for that!"

I went back to my eye doctor to tell him all of my symptoms. He gave me another examination and told me to find a Child Strabismus Eye Surgeon who was willing to do surgery on my left eye muscles. It took me a full year to get an appointment with several eye surgeons and then have the surgery.

Shortly after the surgery, I was back at the surgeon's office. Nothing had changed for me visually and none of my symptoms had changed. I was still stuck in the horror movie that had turned my life upside down. My symptoms were so bad that I begged him to "put horse blinders on the sides of my eyeglass frames" because my brain could not handle using any peripheral vision. He said there wasn't anything else he could do for me and I left his office feeling defeated.

Over the next four years, I went from working in engineering and building products, multitasking on several projects, and running a crew of workers to being a basic wiring harness assembler. I'd left 13 jobs in a fit of fight or flight rage not knowing what was going on with me.  I also had to give up my Commercial Drivers License (CDL-A) and my hobby as a Crew Chief for a drag racing team.

Gone were the days of being creative and spontaneous. Gone were my multi-tasking and high functioning organizational skills. Gone were my incredible hand-eye coordination and visual spatial awareness. Gone was the "old me", but I was going to fight to get any remnants of him back.

When my daughter was about seven years old, I found her sitting on the living room floor flipping through old photo albums. What really caught her attention were pictures of the "old me" doing fun activities with her older brother. She grew up only knowing me as having a brain injury as her older brother knew me before and after the injury. Her normal was having an anxiety-filled, recluse for a father. I could see her anger building as she turned each page. She looked up at me and angrily asked, "When are WE going to do these things?" I told her I was doing everything I could to get back to doing those things and as soon as I figured out what was going on with my vision we would do all of those things and more.

I saw two more providers who diagnosed me with Post Trauma Vision Syndrome and provided me with prism lenses. For some reason, the lenses alone did not work for me. They were very overwhelming to my vision system and were not making a difference.

The code I could not crack was the one that could get my brain to process vision correctly again. Eventually, my visual processing speed slowed down to where I could not even help Veterans and their family members anymore. Like a candle that had flickered in the wind, trying to stay lit for far too long, it finally blew out and I felt like I had lost everything good in my life.

I found myself wishing that the hit to my head had killed me.

As I focused on rehabilitation for my brain injury, my vision problems made it difficult for me to do speech therapy, occupational therapy, and vestibular therapy. During another failed session of speech therapy, my speech therapist yelled at me, "I'm making up cues and you're not even seeing them!"

I was so upset that I went to my Neurologist and demanded, "Give me a referral to anyone who knows anything about the vision problems I'm having!"

Finally, after twelve horrible years, I got the right referral to the right Optometrist who gave me the right neuro-optometric evaluation, prescription lenses with prisms, and a vision therapy treatment plan.

In the meantime, I persevered onward by helping Veterans and athletes with Traumatic Brain Injuries and their family members. They would always tell me, "You're the only one who has given us information about TBI and how to get help for it!"

After an extensive examination, I was diagnosed with Post Trauma Vision Syndrome and visual/vestibular processing imbalance. I was prescribed glasses with prisms and referred to Eye Q Vision Therapy Center for vision therapy.

I asked my eye doctor to provide me with an explanation of the vision problems people can have following a Traumatic Brain Injury. He explained:

*"The symptoms and experiences that Ted describes so vividly, although slightly different in every brain-injured patient, all have a common thread and, a common cause. The vestibular system, which is comprised of a fluid based feedback mechanism located within the inner ear, gives the brain information about acceleration, orientation and the body's location in space. This system needs to coincide with the same type of information being sent to the brain by the visual system as well as through experiences via the proprioceptive or touch system.*

*When there is conflict between what the vestibular, visual and/or proprioceptive systems are sending to the brain, that conflict creates uncertainty, perceived movement of the world and internal nausea or wooziness. Therapy involving only one of these systems by itself does not seem to be as effective as intervention that utilizes vestibular, visual and proprioceptive therapy together to recreate the synchrony that we all take for granted.*

*First, patients may show little or no measurable damage on tests like MRI or CT, but still may still suffer greatly, is a necessary starting point for providers in guiding the proper treatment.*

*Furthermore, understanding that we are built with a bi-modal visual system, is critical. In asymptomatic individuals, the central or focal visual system is balanced and in sync with the ambient or peripheral visual system. Individuals can attend to both central information and peripheral information simultaneously without excessive effort or compromise.*

*They may sacrifice peripheral vision in order to focus on some detail in their central field, causing them to lose the ability to navigate in a straight path or bump into something unknowingly. Movement in the periphery when attending to a central target, such as sunlight through the trees when driving down the road, can overwhelm the system and cause extreme fatigue, dizziness, and nausea. Conversely, they may sacrifice central vision and miss important details when something in their peripheral vision requires their attention.*

*Understanding how these systems operate and the potential effect that often result from trauma is critical in guiding the systems back toward their normal state."*

While I was waiting for my new pair of glasses with prism lenses to come in, I began vision therapy.  It consisted of a combination of Syntonics (Optometric Phototherapy), Dynavision D2, and Computer-Aided Vision Therapy. As soon as I got my new glasses, I walked around the mall with my family members to see if I would have to run out of the place as I had to so many times before. I stopped on the upstairs of the mall and looked around. I then turned around and asked my daughter to take a picture of me with a smile on my face because the prisms were working.

Starting vision therapy and then getting my prism lenses made all the difference in getting my brain's vision processing systems functioning together again. After every vision therapy session, I noticed a positive change in my visual processing. I was amazed that I did not have any bad side effects from the therapy. In fact, the therapy was easy. It was almost too easy.

I had a much-unexpected surprise from the vision therapy! I noticed that I could once again tolerate listening to the radio while driving. Before vision therapy, listening to the radio while driving was overwhelming and impossible because I had an auditory processing disorder as a result of my Traumatic Brain Injury (the same brain injury that caused my vision problems.) I contacted my audiologist at the Manchester VA Medical Center and requested that he retest me to verify if what I had noticed was true.  He agreed to retest me and the test results verified my auditory processing disorder was gone.

I learned that my vision and auditory processing problems were located exactly where I was hit in my right temporal lobe.

> "I had a much-unexpected surprise from the vision therapy! I noticed that I could once again tolerate listening to the radio while driving."

Unfortunately, it didn't take away all of my vision problems. Issues remain such as depth perception and tracking, long-lasting brain injury deficits with executive function, working memory, attention, neuro-fatigue, talking too much, left side weakness and pain, etc., all associated with my damaged right frontal, temporal and parietal lobes.

No longer do I have to leave my family members stranded as I ran out of a grocery store, mall or school because I am in a full-blown panic attack. They no longer have to make excuses for why I'm not at events, because I now can attend all of them. Better still, they don't have to hold onto me to keep me steady on my feet anymore when I stand for the National Anthem.

I have been able to drive to and attend my daughter's dance recitals and sporting events at school, my son's college graduation at Gillette Stadium, a Boston Bruins game at TD Garden, and drag racing at New England Dragway. I've yet to attend a NASCAR race at New Hampshire International Speedway since getting my vision processing back on track, but it's on my list of things to do. I miss taking my family to the races.

I cannot stress enough the importance of getting a proper neuro-optometric evaluation for vision problems after a Traumatic Brain Injury (TBI) and then getting the right lenses and vision therapy (if needed.) You owe it to yourself and your family to pursue this so that you're no longer sitting at home alone on a couch while your family members are out enjoying life. No longer do you have to be far away and left behind!

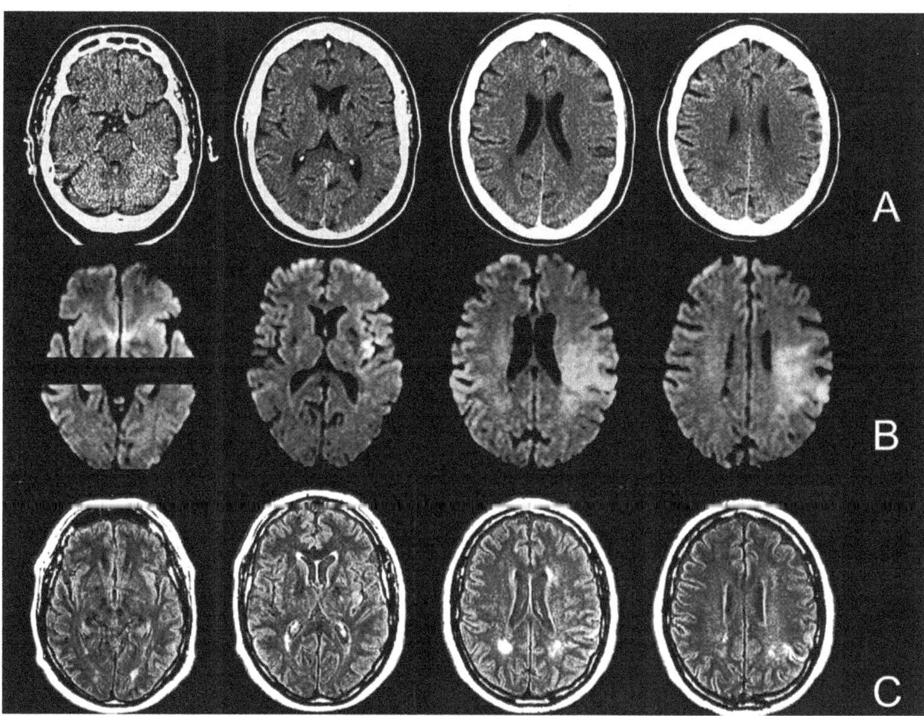

Most TBI survivors do not understand how the brain's vision processing systems work and therefore they do not know how to explain what is happening to them. When they get their vision checked and it is 20/20 (with or without glasses), everyone thinks their vision is fine. They do not understand that even with 20/20 vision they can still have functional vision problems. We are mistakenly taught through television, movies and other media that if something does not show up on an MRI or CT Scan, then there must not be anything wrong with us.

I cannot count the number of times I wished I had the piece of metal sticking out of my head or my left eye still going outward and upward like a sideshow exhibit. Family members, friends, co-workers, teammates and others do not understand what you are going through because it's an *invisible injury*. When it affects you behaviorally, people think you are being over-dramatic, faking or looking for attention.

Nowadays, if I am sitting on the couch, I have my headphones on listening to music, thinking about my brain injury journey, and typing it all out on my laptop computer. My mission is to advocate for Traumatic Brain Injury survivors, their family members, and caregivers by giving them a voice as many of them can't explain what they are experiencing.

It has been four years now since my life changed for the better. I am happy to report that I've driven highways into the White Mountains of New Hampshire, the Green Mountains of Vermont, up the coast of Maine, and into the city of Boston, Massachusetts while happily listening to and singing the song, "Don't Look Back" by the band Boston. I find that rather fitting.

## Meet Ted Stachulski

*Ted Stachulski is a former multi-sport athlete, Marine Corps Veteran, Traumatic Brain Injury Survivor, creator of the Veterans Traumatic Brain Injury Survivor Guide. Ted is also a Veterans Outreach Specialist and an advocate for brain injury survivors, their family members and caregivers. You can learn more about Ted at www.TBITed.com*

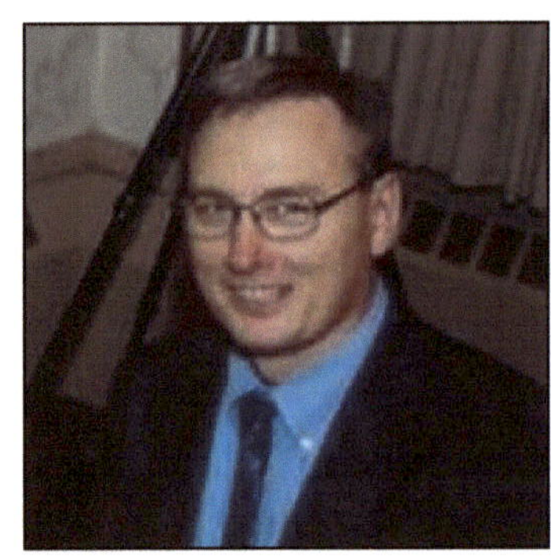

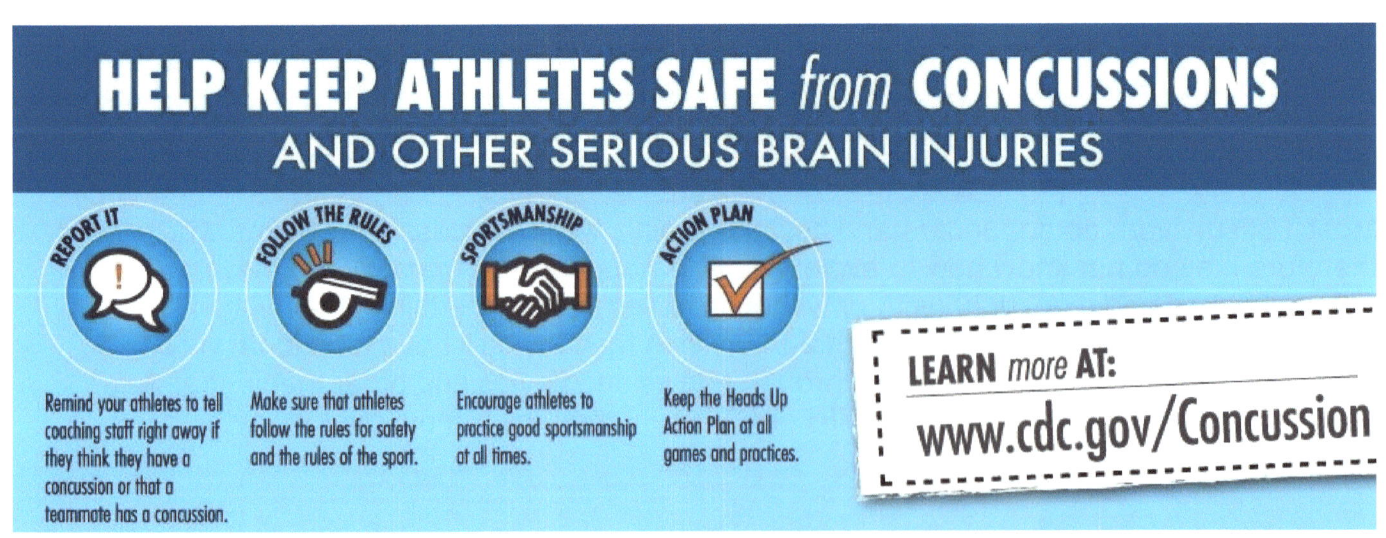

# News & Views

There is nothing that can prepare you for all that comes with life after brain injury. Whether it is an acquired brain injury - like a stroke, or a traumatic brain injury, the net result is that life is forever changed.

Back in 2010, we had our lives changed forever. For a long time, several years in fact, we were unable to visualize what a meaningful life would look like. In fact, for a long time, we thought it to be a virtual impossibility.

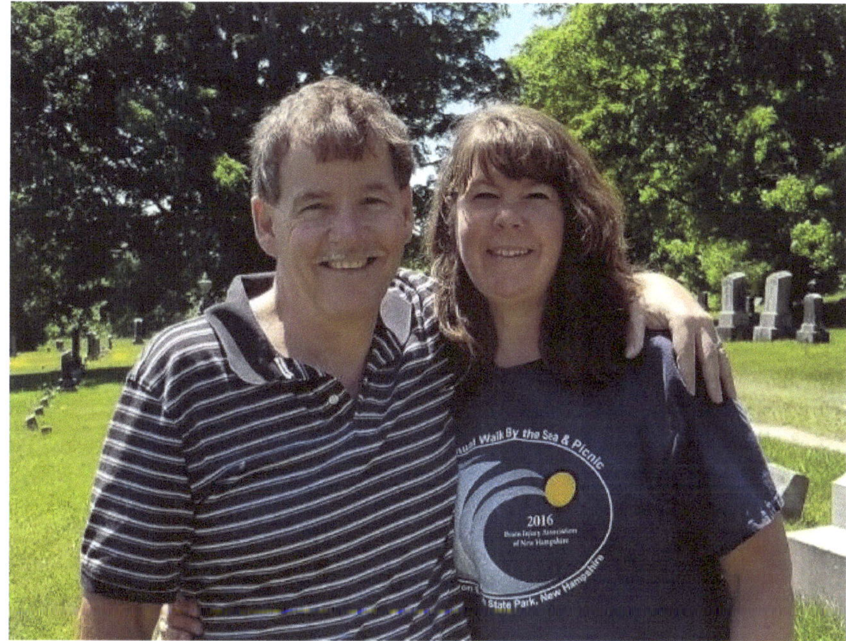

Time has a way of putting things into perspective.  Our lives today are vastly different from anything we could have imagined. Somewhere along the way, both Sarah and I said, "this is not how our story is going to end."

One of our goals with every issue of HOPE Magazine is to share with others the same message – that though brain injury does indeed change everything about life as you know it, a new life can be rebuilt.

This month's contributing writers have walked through seemingly insurmountable adversity, yet today, all of them have found a way to embrace life after brain injury. As anyone with a heartbeat can attest to, there will be times that we all stumble and fall. But with courage and dignity, we get up, brush ourselves off, and move forward.

The common message shared in this issue is that while there are many paths to recovery, life can again become worthwhile, meaningful and rewarding.

We hope you have come away from this month's issue with renewed hope and inspiration.

*~David & Sarah*

www.ingramcontent.com/pod-product-compliance
Lightning Source LLC
Chambersburg PA
CBHW040203240726
48664CB00002B/811